YOGA
FOR
BEGINNERS

Practical Yoga To Improve Your Breathing, Heal Your Body And Balance Your Mind.

Diane Clarke

© 2015

Table Of Contents

1. Introduction

Welcome and thank you for exploring my exciting new book on the science of Yoga!

Yoga is a revered science that has been around for over 5000 years. But today, the Western world is unfortunately more likely to be fed an individual's mickey-mouse version of Yoga, than the pure, authentic science!

Yoga is now seen as a fashionable daily routine to bless ourselves with good health and fitness. While it's truly, absolutely fantastic that Yoga studios have mushroomed all over the world in the past few decades, this has also brought with it its fair share of distortion and misrepresentation of the original science.

Through this book, I re-introduce Yoga from its *original* source.

In this book, I focus on *asanas* (body postures), *pranayama* (breathing practices) and Yoga *mudras* (hand gestures). These three facets of Yoga have gained immense popularity with modern enthusiasts. But in addition to this, I also capture the less known facets of Yoga that together make it the profound, purposeful science it is.

This book is also a *practical* guide to help you kick-start your own profound practice. While the first section provides a background on this marvelous science, the rest of the book is sprinkled with *45 impressive Yogic routines* that can bring your entire mind-body-spirit back to its original harmony.

In this book, you will find:
-Yogic practices to rejuvenate all components of you (body, mind and soul).
-Direct techniques to expand your breath and gain more energy.
-Potent visualization techniques to get more out of your practice.
-Therapeutic postures, breathing techniques and hand gestures to:
-Balance diabetes.
-Overcome heart disorders and balance your blood pressure.
-Improve your metabolism and fix your digestion.
-Beat long standing obesity and trigger permanent weight loss.
-Strengthen your back and heal pain.

I urge you to try them all; if possible, with supervision. The poses captured here are *SAFE* and can be comfortably practiced by beginners. But when you engage with an experienced teacher, you can learn to better tune your body and your mind to this holistic science.

In the final chapter called "Next Steps", I've outlined profound Yoga programs that can raise your practice to the next phenomenal level. I encourage you to explore them and find your unique path to Yogic nirvana.

With this, I wish you extraordinary success in the powerful journey ahead!

~ Diane Clarke

SECTION – 1

REINTRODUCING YOGA

1. What Is Yoga

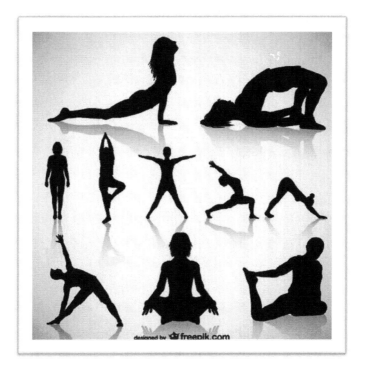

First up, let me assure you that this first section is the only one that is heavy with theory!

But I believe that for us to be suitably impressed with any new practice, we must recognize the integrity and completeness of the science behind it. Once we are convinced, we will willingly commit to it for the long haul.

Through this chapter, you will discover the subtle and varied forms that Yoga tries to use to direct us inwards to our *true* self. This knowledge will help you realize the sheer depth of this science, and hence initiate a successful practice.

With this, I now re-introduce the science of Yoga to you.

YOGA IS:
Not just a fitness routine!
Yoga is not a mere fitness routine that includes physical postures and breathing

exercises. Yoga is a clear, complete *science* that was revealed to a *Vedic* Enlightened Master, Patanjali.

Its goal was lofty and absolute: *to help man reach his ULTIMATE self!*

In Vedic tradition, we call this state *"Advaitha"* or *"Nirvikalpa"*. In Western tradition, we call this "Enlightenment". Today, we recognize this as manifesting the highest possibility of ourselves!

Yoga is also intended to be a sincere and authentic *practice*. Yoga must make us more flexible each day, in our body AND in our mind. This does not mean that we have to turn ourselves into a pretzel! But Yoga will empower us to fully open up our body and mind, and to our own boundless possibilities.

An inclusive science!

Contrary to popular notion, the practice of Yoga does not force us to give up life's possibilities. From food habits to lifestyle, from mental patterns to consciousness, it includes them all and helps us achieve the ultimate by transcending low-level possibilities.

It works on the underlying harmony in this universe that is also reflected within all parts of our system: breath, mind, body and soul, AND our connection with everything around us. Each facet of Yoga is cleverly derived from the dynamics between these different parts, and helps us discover higher and more powerful dimensions of our own self.

A "PURE" science

The original science is called *Patanjali* Yoga. This is also called *Ashtanga* Yoga, referring to the eightfold path of this science. From this is *Hatha* Yoga, which deals with *asanas* or physical Yogic poses to achieve balance. *Iyengar* Yoga specifically aligns to this science, and was popularized by B.K.S Iyengar who initiated a major revival of this form in the 20th century.

All other forms of Yoga – *Power* Yoga, *Hot* Yoga, *Kundalini* Yoga, *Acro* Yoga, *Prenatal* Yoga, *Restorative* Yoga, *Bikram* Yoga, *Anusara* Yoga, *Yin* Yoga, etc. are essentially isolated forms endorsed by individuals or sects that are not part of the original source.

I'm not saying that these other forms do not help. Yoga is a voluminous science and isolating even a part of it for practice still brings profound benefit. But imagine that you have varied forms of your chosen faith: Power Christianity, Yin Buddhism, Acro Hinduism, Prenatal Judaism or Hot Islam? I'm pretty sure you'd prefer the *original* source.

It's the same with Yoga.

Whatever is your need to pursue Yoga (from mild curiosity, to gain peak health and fitness, as a fashionable lifestyle to achieve balance and clarity, et.), I urge you to seek a teacher who has also studied the *original, untainted* science that has withstood over 5,000 years of life-altering change. You're worth it!

Benefits of practicing Yoga

Yoga is not just a casual lifestyle practice, but a profound way of life. Every facet and limb of Yoga is intended to benefit man, and raise him to his highest possibility.

Here, I outline the top 4 benefits of adapting a Yogic lifestyle.

Awaken your Kundalini energy: If you think you're currently "alive", just wait until your Kundalini is awakened! This is the *dormant* life force energy that lies in every human being. When awakened through Yoga, we enjoy enormous creativity, fearlessness and courage, clarity of thought and are showered in gratitude.

Restore physical, mental, emotional and spiritual health: The Yogic principle of treating any disease as simple lack of ease makes it straightforward to restore health. For every disorder, there is a healing Yogic routine to initiate the journey back to health and harmony.

Enhance concentration and productivity: Yoga trains our mind to let go of its inherent need to wander. We intensely focus on the present. We enjoy increased concentration and productivity.

Raise our perception of ourselves: This is the most subtle yet powerful benefit of Yoga. Yoga has to be embraced as an expansive way of *living* that helps raise our awareness. We no longer feel confined by our limiting beliefs and ideas and become easily open to higher possibilities.

2. An Eightfold Path

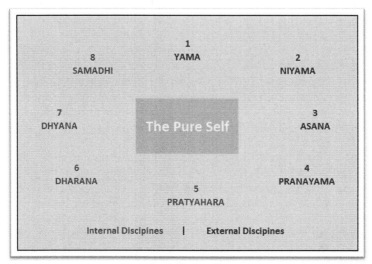

1: The 8 Limbs of Yoga

Yoga recognizes that man is primarily made up of 2 elements:

Pure consciousness *(purusha):* This is *whole, living energy,* and encompasses everything that exists.

Matter *(prakriti):* This is the *fragmented* part of ourselves that we mistakenly believe defines us. Due to our ignorance, we attribute ourselves to this gross matter (includes the body, mind, thoughts, beliefs and ideas that stem from past experiences).

Matter is only a superficial veil covering pure consciousness. Yoga is a fool-proof journey to achieve union with this pure consciousness.

Patanjali, the founder of Yoga spread the entire science into 8 parts. The first four paths are *external disciplines*, and effective recommendations on how we can conduct ourselves with the external world to achieve inner harmony. The next four paths are *internal disciplines*, and take us deeper into this harmony.

The deeper is the path, the more subtle its practice!

I have provided a brief introduction to each path below. As you will see, these paths require resilience and are not for the faint-hearted. It is no wonder that the larger part of the world has satisfied itself with using mere postures and breathing techniques as convenient methods to achieve balance!

In this section, I hope for you to have at least a glimpse of the larger science.

1.Yama (Social conduct)
This branch teaches us the best way to externally conduct ourselves with society, and is based on the following 5 virtues:
-Non-violence (*ahimsa*) in life.
-Truthfulness (*satya*) with self and others.
-Non-stealing (*asteya*) from others.
-Celibacy (*brahmacharya*) in body, mind and spirit until marriage, and for those who seek the renunciate's path.
-Non-accumulation of things (*aparigraha*) that aren't truly required in our life. This teaches us to live a life of simplicity and non-possessiveness.

2. Niyama (Personal conduct)
This branch teaches us to function from the following 5 virtues:
-Purity (*shaucha*) in the mind and body.
-Complete contentment (*santosha*), with ourselves, others and all aspects of our lives.
-Tapa (*austerities*) to strengthen ourselves.
-Thorough self-study (*svadhyaya*).
-Total surrender (*ishvarapranidhan*) to the divinity within and around us.

3. Asana (Yogic body postures)
This is perhaps the most popular practice of Yoga, and is the key ingredient to achieve optimum physical health and fitness. Each posture works on the science of your body's anatomy, with each pose providing a gentle massage to your *internal* organs. It is for this reason that *asanas* are also used for physical healing and restoration.

4. Pranayama (Expansion of breath)
Yoga ascertains that it is not just our breath that gives life to us, but our consumption of the life-force energy (*prana*) through our breath which determines the amount of life and energy we *exude*. Yoga is also clear that our breath is a direct reflection of the state of our mind and body. The more chaotic or shallow is our breathing, the more conflicted we are in body and mind. Through *pranayama*, we can regularize and expand our breath to bring our body and mind to instant harmony.

5. Pratyahara (Withdrawal of our five senses)
We're slowly heading towards more subtle Yogic practices.

By nature, our senses constantly seek fulfillment through external pleasures. Our tongues feast on flavor, our ears enjoy music, our eyes cherish beauty, our noses loves fragrance, and our skin craves touch. These are all external stimuli, directed at (dead) *matter*.

But through *pratyahara*, all our externally tuned senses are slowly taught to turn "inward", towards pure, *living*, consciousness.

The term "withdrawal" should not be misunderstood, as no part of Yoga advocates self-denial! Instead, the practice of *pratyahara* multiples your capacity for fulfillment, as this is now driven by living energy (instead of dead matter).

6. *Dharana* (concentration)
With *dharana* or concentration, our mind is slowly but deliberately trained to focus on the inside, towards meditation. This is a subtle step to *prepare* us for successful meditation.

7. *Dhyana* (meditation)
As you can see, meditation is but one step away from our ultimate goal: Enlightenment. Is it any wonder that the modern world is quite confused about meditation, considering we jump into it with almost no preparation?

In meditation, Yoga teaches us to focus completely on the inside, with no distractions. Again, this is not from denial, but happens as a natural process of our preparation. In meditation, we prepare ourselves for *Samadhi*, spiritual liberation from the bondage of our body, mind and identity.

8. *Samadhi* (Enlightenment)
With steady meditation, we are effortlessly able to stay for longer periods in the "no-mind" state, where we are not bound by our thoughts or our limited identity. When we are powerfully established in this state, we are in *Samadhi*, the final journey towards Enlightenment. There are several levels of *Samadhi*, each reflecting our state of conscious evolution. With *nirvikalpa* (the final stage), we rise above gross matter, and merge into pure consciousness. We become willingly Enlightened!

3. Getting started

I bet you're super eager to kick-start your Yogic practice. We will, real soon!

In this book, I'm going to constrain "Yogic practice" to mean the practice of *asanas* (body postures), *pranayama* (breathing practices) and Yoga *mudras* (hand gestures). But you have now additional knowledge to go into deeper practices.

Guidelines for *effective* practice

-*Embrace your Yoga mat, literally:* Your practice will rewire your Yoga mat with your (evolving) bio blueprint. You'll also find yourself often drawn to your mat to practice deeper techniques. But do avoid sharing your mat with others to keep external interference from ruining your evolving bio blueprint!

-*Hydrate, "adequately":* Some folks go through an entire bottle of water during a 1-hour session. This is simply not necessary, and can interfere with breathing techniques towards the end of the session. Yoga rejuvenates you inside out, so your body is replenished with anything it loses during the session. As a beginner, you can choose to sip on water until you feel comfortable.

-*Timing:* For beginners, Yoga is best practiced on an empty stomach or at least 4 hours after a meal. With time, you will find your metabolism dramatically improve so you can start a routine within a couple of hours after a meal.

-*Warm-up*: Begin your session with a good warm-up; only then will you get a good stretch during your session. You can try the rousing "*Patanjali Dhyaan*," where we imagine our entire body to be made of 5 separate snakes:
-Our 2 arms
-Our 2 legs
-Our neck and head region
-For a graceful yet invigorating warm-up, move those 5 snakes like they're *dancing,* to their own individual rhythm. This is an awesome, playful warm-up routine that will leave you feeling energized in minutes. Begin with 1 minute and extend to 3-5 minutes.

-*Order:* The best order for your Yoga practice is as follows:
-*Warm-up* -> *Asana* -> *Pranayama* -> *Kriya* -> *Meditation* (with *mudra*s)

-*Breathe*: This is the key to a fantastic, energizing session! Pace your inhale with upward movement and exhale with downward or shrinking movement. Tune your breath to suit your posture and watch how vibrant you feel at the end of your session!

-Visualize: Often, your mind interferes with your routine.
-Oh this posture is tooo hard!
-I surely can't stretch that much! I'm not that flexible!
-As your mind wills, your body moves. But with Yoga, you can bend your body, and your mind! Begin a difficult routine with visualization as you imagine yourself *effortlessly* executing it. Do this for a good minute. Then, before your mind can interfere again, pounce on your posture. JUST DO IT! Even if you don't execute it with 100% flexibility, you will still execute it much better than your initial doubts allowed you to believe.

-Stability and comfort: These are the two traits of any successful posture. Stretch/ bend/ jump/ move only up to the limit of your comfort level.

-Readiness: If you're recovering from injury, surgery or are pregnant, you are strongly advised to consult with your physician before beginning your practice!

Ujjayi breath

At this point, I'm going to introduce you to a powerful new breathing technique called, "*Ujjayi* breath". We typically inhale through the nose. Here, we use the *throat region* to expand the breath.

When you first take up Yoga, you may notice that your shallow breathing does not last long enough to support your posture and can ruin the rhythm of your practice as your breath goes out of sync with the posture. *Ujjayi* breath helps you expand your breath to suit your posture.

Instructions:
1. Sit straight and focus your attention on your throat region. Slowly inhale, using your nose and *throat* (without force). Hold for just 1-2 seconds.
2. Exhale using your throat and hold for 1-2 seconds.
3. One trick is to *gently* tighten the epiglottis at the center of your throat during inhale. Put gentle pressure, without restricting your inhalation; you should have a *longer* inhale. Release this pressure slowly for a longer exhale.
4. Do this for 8-10 breaths, until you get the hang of it.
Don't stress too much about it, as this is a safe, effortless technique that will come with practice. When you're doing it right, you should sound like Darth Vader, straight out of Star Wars! ☺

Your first Yogic posture!

1.   Padahastasana
(Gorilla pose)

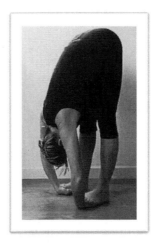

Instructions:
1. Stand straight with your feet 6 inches apart and arms loosely by the side. This is called "*samasthiti*" or *Tadasana*, a common root posture for most Yogasanas. Find balance (comfort and stability) in this posture.
2. Inhale with *Ujjayi* breath and stretch your arms above your head and close to your ears.
3. Exhale with *Ujjayi* breath and bend down *from your hip* to touch your toes. Ensure that your back and knees remain straight.
4. Now hold your feet in each arm, or place your palms flat in front of your feet. (Beginners can reach as close to your toes as possible).
5. You are now in *Padahastasana;* breathe normally and hold this for 4-8 breaths.
6. Retrace your path: inhale, rise and stretch your arms above your head.
7. Exhale and come back to *samasthiti*.

Repetitions: 3 sets, slowly increasing the hold time to 10-30 breaths. Visualize the posture before each repetition.

Benefits:
Removes *tamas*, the inertia or physical laziness in us. This posture is hence executed as the first routine in a session.
Stretches the whole body and makes it more flexible.
Stretches the back and hamstring muscles
Massages digestive organs and intestinal muscles and regularizes their functions
Improves blood circulation even as the brain gets a welcome dose of invigorating energy!

You might wonder why I've taken up a whole page to describe this very simple posture. This is to help you embrace some simple techniques for a more enjoyable practice.

-Comfort and stability in *samasthiti* (or your root posture): This will lead to better balance during the rest of the pose.
-Correct and *straight* posture (with erect spine, neck and head) at all times.
-Visualization: Use this each time you feel you aren't getting a good stretch. You will find the next repetition better!
-Bend from the hip for a more effective stretch.
-*Ujjayi* breathing to extend your breath and sync it with each posture: Whether you desire health, fitness, weight loss or stress relief, the more *mindful* your Yogic practice is, the better the results. Hence, remember to constantly use your breath to pace your posture, stay mindful, avoid boredom and have FUN!

SECTION - 2

ROARING INTO YOUR YOGA PRACTICE!

4. Yoga for the Mind

You might wonder why we're beginning our full scale Yoga practice with the mind and not the body. We WILL practice *asanas* or body postures here. But we will first remove all mental restlessness and instability, annoying disturbances that can disrupt your practice.

All postures outlined in this chapter quell restlessness and calm the mind. These techniques can also be practiced in isolation or anytime you're feeling stressed or unsettled. Together, they can seamlessly bring you back to balance.

For absolute beginners who struggle with poor stamina and flexibility, the exercises outlined in this chapter are enough to make up the first few sessions or your practice. As you progress, you can move to more advanced postures.

2.   Uttanasana

(Standing forward bend pose)

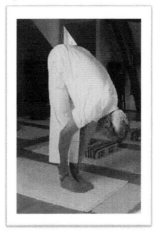

Instructions:
1. Come to *samasthiti*.
2. Inhale and raise your arms up above your head. Stretch as much as possible, and breathe normally for 1-2 seconds.
3. Exhale and bend down *from your hip* to touch your toes.
4. Now hold your (lower) calf muscles and gently lower your forehead so it is as close to your knees as possible. Your spine and knees should remain erect.
5. You are now in *Uttanasana,* a gentle, relaxing posture; breathe normally and hold this for 10-12 breaths to enjoy its calming effect.
6. Retrace your path. Inhale and stretch up, lifting your arms above your head.
7. Exhale and come back to *samasthiti*.

Repetitions: 3 sets, gently increasing the hold time to 20-30 seconds.

Benefits:
Easier variant of *Padahastasana*; often used to open a beginner's class.
Combats fatigue, depression, low moods, nervousness and anxiety.
Improves flexibility.
Soothe the mind.
The longer you can hold the posture, greater the benefits!

Contraindications:
Do NOT practice this is you have slip disk, varicose veins or recent (back) injury.

3. Trikonasana
(Triangle pose)

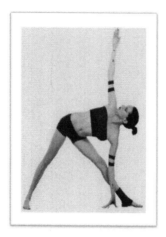

Instructions:
1. Come to *samasthiti*. Move your legs wide apart and parallel to each other.
2. Move your right foot (by 90°), so it turns right. Also move your left foot by 15° so it faces your right foot.
3. Inhale and raise your arms from the side to shoulder height, palms facing the ground. Your arms should be parallel to the ground.
4. Press your right foot, exerting slight pressure and find your balance.
5. As you exhale, bend your entire body to your right and place your right palm on the ground in front of your right foot. Look up at your left palm.
6. You are in *Trikonasana;* keep your knee and spine erect and breathe normally while you hold this for 4-8 breaths. (Beginners can place their forearms on their right thigh.)
7. Inhale and raise yourself so your arms are at shoulder length and parallel the ground.
8. Exhale and come back to *samasthiti*.

Repetitions: 3 sets on each leg.

Benefits:
Balancing pose; excellent to diffuse stress and anxiety.
Opens up stiff hips and strengthens legs and calf muscles.
Improves digestion.
Helps relieve leg and sciatica pain.

Contraindications:
Do NOT practice this is you have migraine or blood pressure problems.

4. Vrikshasana

(Tree pose)

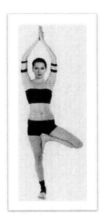

Instructions:
1. Come to *samasthiti*.
2. Lift your right leg, and place it flat on top of your left thigh. (Beginners can place their leg on the left knee and work their way up with practice.)
3. Inhale and gently lift your arms up from the side, and join your palms together above your head, (in the welcoming Namaskara *Mudra*).
4. You are in *Vrikshasana;* breathe normally and hold this for 4-8 breaths.
5. Exhale and bring your arms back to your side, gently lowering your leg to the ground.

Tip:
To find better balance for any posture, focus your eyes at a point 1-2 feet away from you. By keeping your attention steady on this point, you can remain in balance throughout the posture.

Repetitions: 3 sets on each leg.

Benefits:
Quells restlessness and improves physical and mental balance.
Improves focus and concentration.
Strengthens legs and calf muscles. Recommended for those suffering from sciatica pain.

Contraindications:
Do NOT practice this if you struggle with insomnia, blood pressure problems or migraine.

5. Garudasana
(Eagle pose)

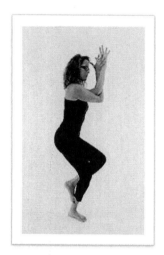

Instructions:
1. Come to *samasthiti*. Focus on a point and find your balance.
2. Inhale as you do the following:
a. Bend your right knee, raise your leg and cross it over your left calf.
b. Tuck your right toes behind your left leg.
3. Keep your back straight and your right toes pointed down.
4. Exhale as you do the following:
a. Bend your elbows and gently raise your arms in front and parallel to your face.
b. Bring them close and cross your left arm over your right arm (from the inside)
5. Let your palms face each other. You are in *Garudasana*; breathe normally and hold this for 4-8 breaths.
6. Inhale as you release your hands.
7. Exhale as you release your right leg and come to *samasthiti*.

Repetitions: 3 sets on each leg.

Benefits:
Improves posture and brings physical and mental balance.
Stretches and strengthens your forearms, back and calf muscles.

Contraindications:
This posture puts your body weight on your knee. Do NOT practice this is you're recovering from any injury.

6.   Chakravakasana
(Cat-cow stretch)

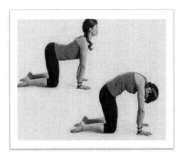

In this pose, you are introduced to *"Vinyasa,"* a facet of Yoga that helps you experience a set of Yoga poses as one, harmonious, flowing dance!

Instructions:
1. Kneel down your mat with your legs a foot apart.
2. Place your arms in front of your legs and lean forward so you're balancing on all fours. Let your heels remain pointed out and up.
3. Your arms should be below your shoulder and your feet should be below your hips even as your neck, head and spine remain erect. Find balance in this posture.
4. Inhale as you get into the *cow pose* – gently drop your stomach down and raise your hips and tailbone high. Arch your back up even as you lift your chest, neck and chin to look up at the sky. Breathe normally for 4-8 seconds.
5. Exhale slowly as you get into the *cat pose* – lift your stomach region up, your tailbone down, and bend your chest, neck and chin to look down. Here, you should look like a cat getting a good, luxurious stretch! Breathe normally for 4-8 seconds.
6. Inhale and gently curve your chin, chest, back and tailbone so you're back in *cow pose*. Hold this for 4-8 seconds. Exhale and slowly stretch back to *cat pose* and hold for 4-8 seconds.
7. Continue to gracefully stretch between the cow and cat pose at least 4 more times. This harmonious dance is *Vinyasa*.

Repetitions: 5-8 sets holding for 4-8 breaths each.

Benefits:
Great warm-up pose to get ready for a more intensive routine.
Can be practiced to re-energize yourself midway through a session.
Increases flexibility, awareness and inner harmony.

Contraindications:
Do NOT practice this is you have slip disk or are recovering from back injury.

7.   Paschimottasana
(Seated forward bend pose)

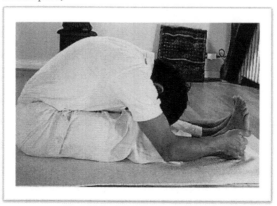

Instructions:
1. Sit straight with your legs together and stretched forward (toes pointing up at the sky). This pose is called *Dandasana* (staff pose).
2. Inhale and stretch your arms above your head.
3. Exhale as bend from the hip and stretch your arms forward towards your toes.
4. Gently lower your head as close to your knees as possible and hold your feet.
5. You are in *Paschimottasana*; breathe normally and hold this for 4-8 breaths. (Beginners can stretch forward as close to the toes as possible).
6. Inhale and raise your back straight slowly, bringing your arms above your head.
7. Exhale and bring your arms back to your side, to *Dandasana*.

Repetitions: 3 sets.

Benefits:
Stretches and strengthens your back.
Massages your abdomen and stomach muscles to improve digestive functions.
Great for weight loss!

8.   Setu Bandhasana
(Bridge pose)

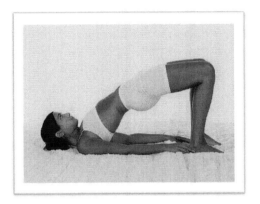

Instructions:
1. Lie down on your back with your legs spread a few inches apart for balance. Your arms should be comfortably placed beside you, palms facing down.
2. Bend your knees and bring your feet towards your tailbone, as close as possible without straining your knees. Find balance in this posture with your head, palms and knees resting firmly and pressed to the ground.
3. Inhale and gently lift your tailbone up so your back is raised above the ground. The higher you can raise your tailbone, the more effective the posture. But do this without strain (especially on your knees and back).
4. You are in *Sethu Bandhasana*; breathe normally and hold this for 4-8 breaths.
5. Exhale as you gently lower your tailbone back to the mat.
6. Repeat this pose 2 times, increasing the hold time to 10 and 15 seconds. With practice, you can keep this posture for up to 30 seconds.

Repetitions: 3-5 sets.

Benefits:
Awesome routine to strengthen the back.
Improves blood circulation.
Improves digestion.

Contraindications:
Do NOT practice this is you are recuperating from back or knee injury.

5. Yoga for the Body

In this chapter, we will slowly step up the scale of the postures involved. Remember to pace your stretch as per your comfort level. Every day, you can aim to lengthen your stretch by ½ an inch more, and extend your pose for a couple of seconds longer.

9.   Utkatasana
(Chair pose)

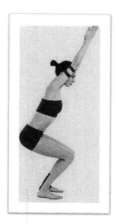

Instructions:
1. Come to *samasthiti*. Spread your feet 6 inches apart.
2. Inhale and raise your arms above your head. Let your palms face each other.
3. As you exhale, bend your knees and slowly squat to sit on an (imaginary) chair. Keep your spine firmly erect.
4. You are in *Utkatasana*; breathe normally and hold this for 6-12 breaths.
5. Inhale and raise yourself back to standing position.
6. Exhale and come back to *samasthiti*.

Repetitions: 3 sets.

Benefits:
Strengthens your spine and your entire leg (calf, thighs, knees).
Improves will power.

Contraindications:
Do NOT practice this if you suffer from migraine, headache, insomnia, knee/ankle injury or arthritis.
Go slow on this pose during your menstrual cycle, or avoid it altogether during this time.

10. Veerabhadrasana
(Warrior pose)

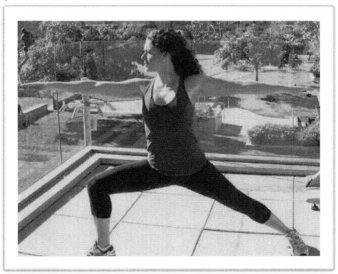

Instructions:
1. Come to *samasthiti*. Move your legs wide apart with your feet parallel to each other.
2. Move your right foot (by 90°), so it faces outside. Move your left foot by 45° so it faces your right foot. Press your right foot, exerting slight pressure and find your balance.
3. Inhale and raise your arms from the side to shoulder height, palms facing the ground. Your arms should be parallel to the ground.
4. Turn your head. Exhale as bend your knees, squat and lean forward to the right.
5. You are in *Veerabhadrasana*. Breathe normally and hold this for 4-8 breaths.
6. Inhale, straighten your knee and come up.
7. Exhale, straighten your head and bring your arms back to your side

Repetitions: 3 sets on each leg.

Benefits:
Strengthens your arms and legs and improves your stamina.
Instills courage, and tangibly improves your confidence.

Contraindications:
Do NOT practice this is you have high blood pressure.

11. Utthita Parshvakonasana

(Extended side angle pose)

While it does sounds like a mouthful, this pose is a powerful, strengthening pose you can easily extend from *Veerabhadrasana*.

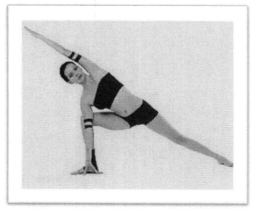

Instructions:

1. From *Veerabhadrasana*, turn your head straight so you are facing forward. You should have your right knee bent, back straight and body pushed downward, and your arms raised to the side, at shoulder height. Breathe normally for 2 seconds.

2. Exhale and gently lower your right palm to the floor, in front of your right foot. (Beginners can place your right forearm on your right thigh.) Find your balance and stay in this posture for 2-4 breaths.

3. Inhale and raise your left hand above your head to form a single, seamless straight line with your left leg.

4. You are in *Utthita Parshvakonasana*; breathe normally and hold this for 4-8 breaths.

5. Inhale and bring your arms back to shoulder height.

6. Exhale and straighten your right knee. Bring your arms back to your side.

Repetitions: 3 sets on each leg.

Benefits:
Strengthens lower back and legs.
Helps with sciatica pain and osteoporosis.

Contraindications:
Do NOT practice this is you have heart problems (like high blood pressure), headache or insomnia.

12. Vajrasana
(Diamond pose)

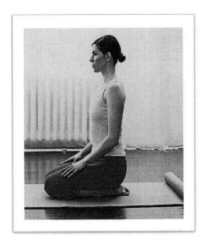

Instructions:
1. Sit on your mat on your heels. Let your tailbone rest on the top of your heels.
2. Keep your spine, neck and head erect and place your palms (facing down) on each thigh.
3. Breathe slowly and observe your breath for 1-2 minutes.

Repetitions: For 15 minutes a day with your favorite *mudra*.

Benefits:
Improves physical and mental balance.
Aids digestion, reduces flatulence and cures constipation.
Improves overall blood circulation.

Contraindications:
This is an incredibly simple pose that is often the root posture for more advanced techniques. However, it does require some flexibility and strong/flexible ankles.
For beginners, you can place a cushion below your ankles or roll up your Yoga mat to support your ankles. With steady practice, you can aim to hold this posture for 5-15 minutes a day (without props) for maximum benefit.

13. Virasana
(Hero pose)

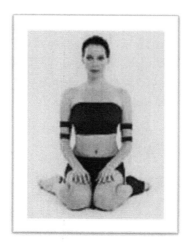

Instructions:
1. Sit comfortably in *Vajrasana*, balanced on your heels.
2. Now gently spread your ankles from below your tailbone, so each ankle rests on either side of your thigh.
3. Keep your spine, neck and head erect and place your palms (facing down) on each thigh.
4. Breathe slowly and observe your breath for 1-2 minutes.

Repetitions: 5-15 minutes a day.

Benefits:
Combines all the benefits of *Vajrasana*
Strengthens feet and improves posture; recommended for those with flat foot.
Benefits arthritis patients

Contraindications:
This is a more advanced pose, and requires strength and flexibility in your ankles and knees.

14. Gomukhasana
(Cow head pose)

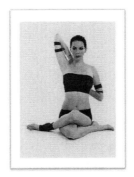

Instructions:
1. Sit straight on your Yoga mat, with your legs together and stretched forward in *Dandasana* (Staff pose).
2. Start with your right leg.
Bend and your right knee and cross your right leg *below* your left thigh.
Bend and lift your left knee and cross your left leg *above* your right thigh.
3. Place your palms on either side of your matt and find balance in this posture.
4. Now for the arms:
   a. Bend your right elbow and raise it *above* your shoulder.
   b. Bend your left elbow and lower it behind your back.
c. Now stretch your arms and clasp them together. If your flexibility doesn't allow this, rest them on your back, as close to each other as possible
5. You are in *Gomukhasana*; breathe normally and hold this for 4-6 breaths.
6. Gently release your hands.
7. Gently uncross your legs, releasing the left foot and then the right.
8. Come back to *Dandasana*, your root posture.

Repetitions: 3 sets on each leg.

Benefits:
An intermediate pose that is excellent for your body and mind.
Improves flexibility, regularizes kidney functions, massages the reproductive organs, strengthens the back and triggers relaxation.
With practice, you can train to hold this posture and breathe normally for up to 20-30 seconds.

Contraindications:
Do NOT practice this is you have had knee injury, or suffer from piles.

15. Navasana
(Boat pose)

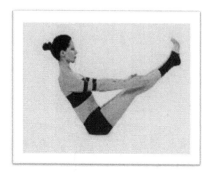

Instructions:
1. Sit straight on your Yoga mat, with your legs together and stretched forward in *Dandasana* (Staff pose).   Find balance in this posture.
2. Lean back slightly (just enough to stretch your back).
3. Focus your awareness at a point straight ahead of you. Keep your eyes on this point through this posture to retain stability and balance.
4. Now tighten your core, straighten your knees and lift your feet UP in the air. Keep them at least 2 feet above the ground.
5. You can place your hands on your thighs/knees for support, without exerting your back. Try and keep your back and knees as straight as possible.
6. If you're doing this right, you should feel its effect at your core, as your abdomen is tightened and strengthened.
7. You are in *Navasana*; breathe normally and hold this for 4-8 breaths.
8. Gently lower your legs. Gently straighten your back. End with a long, deep breath!

This seemingly simple posture is actually an advanced pose. But it's a miracle worker for your core and digestive organs. I've included this as the last of your active workout, and hope that you will soon find the balance and flexibility to enjoy this posture. Good luck!

Repetitions: 3 sets.

Benefits:
Enhances digestive functions, regularizes thyroid glands and helps you lose weight. Improve focus and concentration.

Contraindications:
Do NOT practice this is you have back injury, diarrhea, heart disorders or low blood pressure, and during pregnancy or menstruation.

Suryanamaskar (Sun salutation)

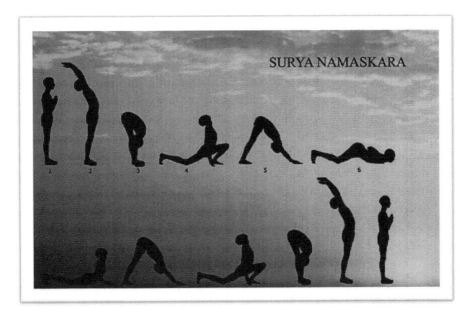

The Suryanamaskar is often revered as the King or Monarch of all Yogasanas!

This is a Vinayasa that comprises a set of 12 synchronized physical postures, each with its own set of amazing benefits, and executed in tandem to one harmonious dance.

With regular practice this can tone up the entire body-mind-spirit system. This is best performed when the sun is out so we can use its energy to rejuvenate ourselves. In fact, Yogic practitioners recommend 24 sets of Suryanamaskar every day to stay active and fit and far away from all physical and mental disease!

Instructions:

16. Pranamasana
(Prayer pose)

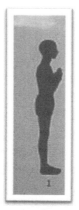

1. Stand straight, with your feet close together.
a. Bring your arms close to your chest, and fold your palms together in salutation (through the welcoming *Namaskara mudra*).

17. Hasta Uttanasana
(Raised arms pose)

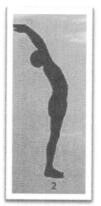

2. *Inhale*, and raise your joined palms up above your head, arching your back backward as you point your (joined) palms to the sky.

18. Pada Hastasana
(Standing forward bend pose)

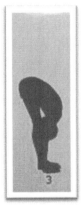

3. Exhale as you bend forward from the hips, and touch your palms to your foot. Knees should stay straight. Beginners can hold the lower calf muscles while flexible folks can hold the bottom of the foot.

19. Ashwa Sanchalanasana
(Equestrian pose)

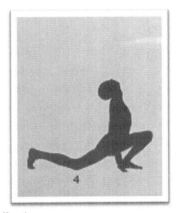

4. Inhale as you do the following:
Stretch the right leg completely backwards, and balance your right leg on your toes. Here, your right knee is bent and heel is raised up.
Bend your left knee.
Raise your head to look up at the sky.
Your palms remain facing downward and rest on your Yoga mat.

20. Adho Mukha Svanasana
(Downward dog pose)

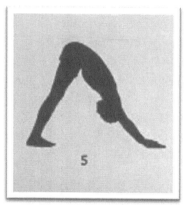

5. *Exhale* and stretch your left knee backwards to join your right leg. Raise your hip up as you look down to the center.

21. Ashtanga Namaskar
(Knees, chest and chin pose)

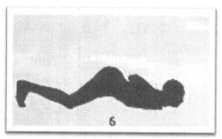

6. *Inhale* as you gently slide down to lie on your stomach. Let your arms rest by either side of your shoulder. *Exhale.*

The actual pose is more advanced, and requires you to slide down with your knees, chest and chin touching the floor even as your hips remain raised and off the floor. Here is the beginner's version.

22. Bhujangasana
(Cobra pose)

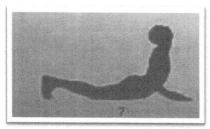

7. Bend your elbows and bring your palms to rest on the mat on either side of your shoulder (to support your weight). *Inhale* and gently lift your chest up from the mat as you arch your back, and look straight. Here, you imitate a cobra with its hood raised and ready to spring, alert and powerful!

23. Adho Mukha Svanasana
(Downward dog pose)

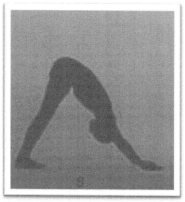

8. *Exhale*, slide down and lift your hips up, to come back to mountain pose.

24. Ashwa Sanchalanasana
(Equestrian pose)

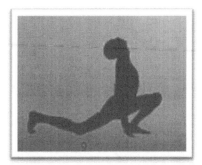

9. *Inhale* as you do the following:

a. Bend your left knee and bring it forward.

b. Balance your right leg on your right toes, with your heel up. Raise your head to look up at the sky.

Your palms remain facing downward, resting on the mat.

25. Pada Hastasana
(Standing forward bend pose)

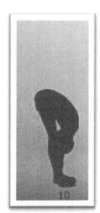

10. *Exhale* as you stand up, hips bent and touch your feet.

26. Hasta Uttanasana
(Raised arms pose)

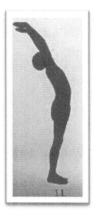

11. Inhale, and stand up fully and raise your joined palms up above your head.

27. Pranamasana
(Prayer pose)

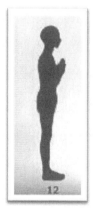

12. Exhale and come back to the root posture, back erect and arms folded and palms joined in front of your chest in a salute (through the welcoming Namaskara *mudra*).

This is one single repetition of the miraculous Suryanamaskar! ☺

Repetitions: 6-24 repetitions on *each* leg.

The Suryanamaskar is an advanced pose. If you're confused or don't get it right the first time, don't get disheartened!

This Yogasana is best learnt from a direct supervisor so you can effortlessly move from pose to pose. However, I place it here for completeness so you will seek to learn it as you begin your practice.

<u>Contraindications</u>:

Do NOT do this if you have any sort of head, neck, back or knee injury!

6. Yoga for the Soul

The modern world can be brutal on our being. Stress, loneliness, depression and isolation are often the unpleasant side-effects of our present lifestyle. In this chapter, you will learn invigorating exercises that help you beat stress, uplift your mood and increase your confidence, and hence easily raise yourself to face life's challenges!

28. Ustrasana
(Camel pose)

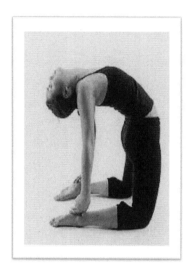

Instructions:
1. Kneel on your yoga mat (using a cushion for beginners). Keep your hands loosely around your hips and find your balance in this posture.
2. Inhale and *gently* bend backwards, stretching your head and your spine, and clasp your heels with your hands. *Attempt this without strain.* Beginners can attempt this pose by placing a pillow or a thick cushion below their knees, to gently ease themselves into this posture.
3. Gently elongate your back and neck, to get a good stretch.
4. You are in *Ustrasana*; breathe normally and hold this for 4-8 breaths.
5. Exhale and gently lift your neck up.
6. Slowly release your hands.

Repetitions: 3 sets.

Benefits:

Helps combat mood swings and depression.
Stretches whole body and improves digestion.
Useful to heal menstrual cramps.

Contraindications:
This is an intermediate pose and requires some flexibility.
Do NOT practice this if you've had a recent injury, neck strain or a stiff back.

29. Balasana

(Child's pose)

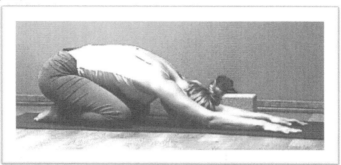

Instructions:
1. Sit in *Vajrasana* supporting your tailbone on your heels. Find balance in this posture.
2. While keeping your tailbone firmly on your heels, exhale and lower your body slowly to rest your forehead on the ground. (Beginners can raise their tailbone slightly to accommodate this.)
3. Now stretch your arms in front of you and place them on the mat, palms facing down.
4. You are in *Balasana*. In this pose, let go of your entire body weight, as if you're letting go of all your worries and stay in this posture for a few minutes.
5. Inhale, and raise yourself back to sitting posture.
6. Exhale, and bring your arms forward. You are back to *Vajrasana*.

Repetitions: 3 sets on each leg.

Benefits:
Excellent to calm down the nervous system!
Relaxes back muscles.
Helps heal constipation.

Contraindications:
Do NOT practice during pregnancy!
Do NOT practice this if recovering from (knee or back) injury.

30. Yoga Mudrasana
(Psychic union pose)

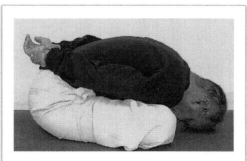

Instructions:
1. Sit in *sukhasana,* with crossed legs.
2. Bring your arms to your back and clasp them. Breathe normally for a few seconds in this posture.
3. With a long exhale, bend your body forward until your forehead touches the ground. For *beginners*, get as close to the ground without straining yourself. You can also lift your hips slightly to help you do this.
4. Relax; you are in *Yoga Mudrasana*. Completely let go and rest in this posture for at least 6-8 seconds.
5. Inhale as come back to *sukhasana* (seated cross-legged pose), while keeping your hands at the back.

Repetitions: 3 sets, slowly extending the hold count to 15-30 seconds.

Benefits:
Awakens the navel center, often the prime indicator of the health of our body-mind system.
Improve digestion and abdominal functions and helps us ingest new and fresh ideas

Contraindications:
Do NOT practice during pregnancy!
Do NOT practice this if recovering from (knee or back) injury or heart related disorders.

31. Makarasana
(Crocodile pose)

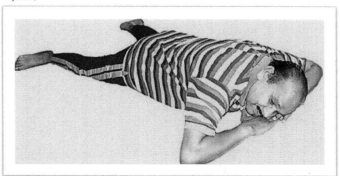

Instructions:
1. Lie down on the mat on your stomach, and cross your arms below your head.
2. Gently rest your head on your arms, and observe your breath.
3. Stretch your legs as you point your toes outwards. If you wish, you can close your eyes.
4. Yep, you are in *Makarasana*! Enjoy this posture breathing normally for 15-20 breaths.

This is a supremely relaxing posture, and is hence practiced either in-between a strenuous session, or towards the end of the session as your body prepares to wind down. This pose is excellent to calm down our nervous system. Any time you feel low, isolated, tired, overwhelmed or lonely, practice this pose.

Repetitions: 3 sets.

Benefits:
Relaxes the body and mind.
Reduces flatulence and abdominal bloating. Helps get rid of constipation.
Relieves back pain.

Contraindications:
Do NOT practice during pregnancy!
Do NOT practice this if recovering from (knee or back) injury.

32. Shavasana
(Corpse pose)

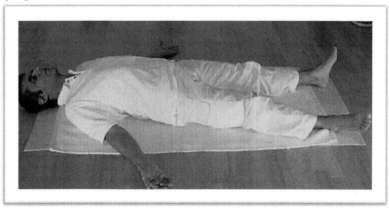

Instructions:
1. Lie down on your back, with your arms by your side (and your palms turned up).
2. Spread your feet about 12-18 inches apart.
3. Just be. Relax; this is the intent of this pose! Stay in this pose for at least 5 minutes, for deep rest and rejuvenation.
4. Sometimes, people tend to doze off in this pose! While this is understandable (especially after a rigorous routine), this is not recommended as the intent of Yoga is to "awaken" you! ☺ Hence, I recommend watching your breath while in *Shavasana*. Alternately, you can start from your feet, and gently connect with every part of your body. You may feel tightness or a subtle tension in certain parts of your body. Continue to observe them while you lie down in *Shavasana* until the tension melts away.

The *Shavasana* is perhaps everyone's favorite "restful" pose, and is hence practiced at the end of an *active* Yoga session. It also provides your body an opportunity to rejuvenate itself after Yoga.

Benefits:
Can cure insomnia and quell physical and mental restlessness.
Shavasana (after a Yoga session) is often recommended to cure depression and fatigue.

7. Yogic breathing: *Pranayama*

Scientists and alternate health practitioners universally agree that most humans use only a small percentage of their lung capacity during breathing.

What causes this? *Shallow breathing*!

It is this incorrect habit that keeps us from making maximum use of our breath, a powerful mechanism to tap into the *life energy* that runs us and this universe.

Most Yogic breathing techniques perform 3 things:
1. Expand our breath and increase the amount of pure life energy or "prana" we consume from air.
2. Powerfully cleanse our body and mind of internal toxins.
3. Increase the heat in our body (unless the technique is captured as an exception).

This reverses a lifetime of incorrect habits and can give your entire system a powerful acid wash!

Notes:
All breathing techniques must be practiced on an empty stomach, or at least 4 hours after a meal.
For beginners, it is best to start your Pranayama practice with a small set of repetitions and build this over time.

Nadi Shodhana Pranayama
(Alternate nostril breathing)
Most of us favor breathing through one nostril more than the other. This reflects an imbalance in our left-brain/ right-brain combination. With this technique, both our nostrils are cleared and optimized for breathing, so we are immediately brought to balance. You will also enjoy a more harmonious left/right brain activity post this technique.

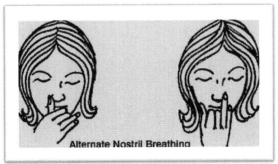

Alternate Nostril Breathing

Instructions:

1. Sit cross-legged or in *Vajrasana* with closed eyes.
2. Keep your left hand on your knee in *Chin mudra (gently press the tips of your thumb and index finger)*. Keep your posture straight.

3. Bring your right hand to your face.
Your *thumb* is placed lightly on your *right* nostril.
Your *ring finger* is placed lightly on your *left* nostril.
Other fingers are held lose.
4. Here, you will alternately inhale and exhale through each nostril.
When you press your thumb, you inhale/ exhale through your left nostril.
When you press your ringer finger, you inhale/ exhale through your right nostril.
Each inhalation and exhalation is *slow and gentle*.
5. You are ready to start!

6. Begin by pressing the thumb, and exhale through the left nostril.
7. Now, practice this technique:
a. Inhale through left nostril. Release thumb.
b. Press ring finger and *Exhale* through right nostril.

c. Inhale through right nostril. Once done, release your ring finger.
d. Press thumb and *Exhale* through left nostril.

e. This is 1 cycle. Repeat 11 repetitions by repeating steps (a) to (d).

Now this may sound confusing. But read the instructions a couple of times and practice with instructions. Soon, you will find the innate harmony in this breathing technique.

<u>Repetitions</u>: 1 set of 11 repetitions (best done early in the morning).

<u>Benefits:</u>
Awesome routine to beat stress and bring mental clarity.
Clears sinus and blocked nose.
Brings us to the present moment, calms the mind and powerfully centers us in reality.

Kapalbhati Pranayama
(Forceful exhalation breathing)
This is an incredibly powerful Yogic-breathing and detoxifying technique. In different traditions, this can also be practiced as Bhastrika.

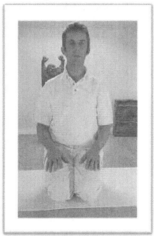

Instructions:
1. Sit cross-legged or in *Vajrasana* or *Sukhasana* (crossed legs) with closed eyes.
2. Keep your hands on your knee or thighs in *Chin mudra (gently press the tips of your thumb and index finger)*. Keep your posture straight.
3. Exhale forcefully, *through your abdomen*. You will physically feel your core tightening with each count of this pranayama. Focus only on your exhalation; your body will automatically inhale as required.
4. Practice this continuously, for 21 forceful exhalations, through your abdomen area.

There's very little a frequent practice of Kapalbhati pranayama cannot do! When you breathe out using the entire force of your abdomen, you push a larger amount of toxins OUT with each exhale, leaving you more pure and powerful, inside. You will notice a pointed difference in your life, before and after regular practice of this technique!

Repetitions: 2-5 sets of 21 repetitions, based on your current fitness.

Benefits:
Dramatically improves your breathing and digestion.
Phenomenal for weight loss.
Improves physical and mental energy levels and combats chronic fatigue.

Contraindications:

Do NOT practice during pregnancy!

Do NOT practice this if recovering from heart related disorders (like high blood pressure).

If you've suffered from chest congestion or back injury, check that it is ok for you to practice this technique.

If you suffer from chronic fatigue or exhaustion, begin this gently as you slowly work your way to a more intensive practice.

33. Bhramari Pranayama
(Humming bee breathing technique)

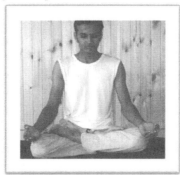

Instructions:
1. Sit cross-legged or in *Vajrasana* with closed eyes. Keep your hands on your knee or thighs in *Chin mudra (gently press the tips of your thumb and index finger).* Keep your posture straight.
2. Bring your attention to your throat and hum like a bumble bee with one long *"hmmmmm"*!
3. Gently inhale, even as you hum. Exhale slowly as you hum. Keep your focus on extending your breath as much as possible even as you hum *without strain.*
4. Practice this continuously for 11 breaths. If this tires you, you can stop after 5-6 breaths, and continue with a second set if possible.

Benefits: This pranayama not only heals your throat center (concerned with your ears, nose and throat) but is also an intensely calming and healing technique. When you find yourself overtly restless, you can practice this technique (on an empty stomach) for a few minutes to get immediate relief and mental clarity. This is also useful to clear headaches and migraines.

Contraindications:
None. However, stop this technique if you feel light-heated or tired.

8. Anytime Yoga: *Mudra* or Hand Gestures

So far, we've explored Yoga as a separate practice, preferably done on an empty stomach on your mat! But what if you could continue with Yoga, any time and at absolutely any place – when you're watching TV, on a phone call, as you walk, etc.?

With Yogic *mudras*, you can!

Mudras are hand gestures that make use of the natural intelligence lying right within the proximity of our fingertips, to trigger profound healing and restorative effects on your body-mind system.

We are the 5 elements!

Yoga clearly understands that every single human being is a divine combination of the 5 elements.

There's more – our hands and feet are a powerful reflection of our entire mind-body-spirit system. We can hence use this knowledge to balance the elements, and bring us to ease and harmony. In Western traditions, we've heard of reflexology. In older eastern traditions, this knowledge is practiced as acupressure and acupuncture techniques. In the ancient Vedic tradition, we tap into this through Yogic *mudras*, or hand gestures.

Finger	Element		Organs	Remarks
Index	Wind	*(VAYU)*	Skin	gaseous, dry
Middle	Space	*(AKASH)*	Ears	subtle
Ring	Water	*(JAL)*	Tongue	flowing, cool
Little	Earth	*(PRITHVI)*	Nose	heavy
Thumb	Fire	*(AGNI)*	Eyes	Powerful!

We use mudras with this knowledge to:
1. Balance an element (by joining the tip of our finger with the tip of our thumb)
2. Increase the presence of an element (by joining the tip of our thumb to the base of the related finger)
3. Decrease the presence of an element (by joining the tip of the related finger to the base of our thumb)
With this, I'm going to quickly introduce you to 10 profound *mudras*, with powerful healing properties.

Notes:

For maximum effect, these *Mudras* can be practiced during Meditation, after 15 minutes of Pranayama. But do remember that these are "anytime" *Mudras*. Hence you can and must practice this every opportunity you get!

Therapeutic *Mudras* can be practiced as follows:

As a single 1-hour session. This will include 45 minutes of therapeutic *mudra* followed by 15 minutes of *Prana mudra*.

In 3 sittings of 20-minute each. This will include 15 minutes of therapeutic *mudra* followed by 5 minutes of *Prana mudra*.

General *mudras* like Jnana/Prana/Apana/Namaskara *mudra* can be practiced for however long you wish.

Practicing *Prana mudra* for 5-15 minutes after any mudra further enhances its strength.

34. Jnana *Mudra*/ Chin *Mudra*

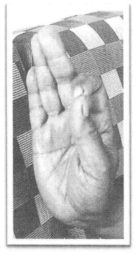

Instructions:
1. Join the tip of your index finger with the tip of your thumb.
2. Hold the remaining 3 fingers straight and lose.
3. Point your palm towards the sky.

Note: When you point your palm towards the earth, this becomes Chin *mudra* (used during Pranayama).

Benefits: This reduces the mental chatter within us and brings about profound transformation *in all levels of our being*! It is hence also called the *Mudra* of (inner) knowledge. At a physical level, it reduces negativity, mental restlessness, heals depression, improves our concentration and balances the air element within us.

Timing: As often and as long as you want!

35. Prana *Mudra*

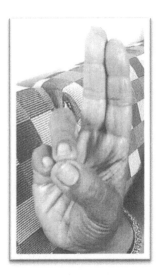

Instructions:
1. Join the tips of your ring and little fingers with the tip of your thumb.
2. Gently hold the remaining 2 fingers straight and lose.

Benefits: This *mudra* is called the *mudra* of "Life Energy". It is hence combined with other healing *mudras* to dramatically increase their beneficial effect. Physically, this *mudra* beats fatigue and invigorates us, heals sinus related problems, improves our immunity and sharpens our eyesight. This also balances the water element within us and cures problems related to water retention (in our body, or in our nose/throat, etc.).

Timing: As often and as long as you want!

36. Apana *Mudra*

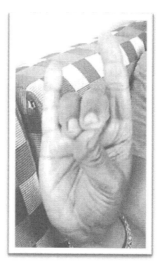

Instructions:
1. Join the tips of your middle and ring fingers with the tip of your thumb.
2. Hold the remaining 2 fingers straight and lose.

Benefits: This *mudra* balances the earth and space elements within us. By doing so, it positively impacts our digestion, and works to effectively *eliminate* all toxins (physical/mental/emotional or spiritual) from our life. This *mudra* can also be used to heal migraine (by practicing Apana *mudra* followed by Jnana *mudra* for 30 minutes each).

Timing: As long as you want! Alternately, you can practice for 45 minutes (followed by 15 minutes of Prana *Mudra*) every day.

37. Vayu *Mudra*

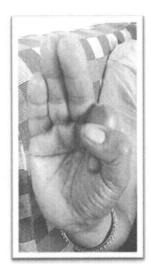

Instructions:
1. Join the tip of your index to the base of your thumb.
2. Gently press your thumb on the back of your index finger.
3. Hold the remaining 3 fingers straight and lose.

Benefits: In Jnana *Mudra*, we reduce excessive air within us. This works wonders to reduce flatulence, *and* unnecessary thoughts! This *mudra* also reduces body pain caused by gas.

Timing: Practice this for 15-45 minutes every day (followed by 5-15 minutes of Prana *mudra*), until the disease is cured.

38. Apana Vayu *Mudra*

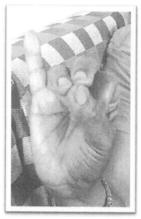

Instructions:
1. This is practiced by combining Apana *mudra* and Vayu *mudra*.
2. Join the tip of your index finger to the base of your thumb.
3. Gently press your thumb on the back of your index finger.
4. Additionally join the tips of your middle and ring fingers with the tip of your thumb.
5. Hold the little finger straight and lose.

Benefits: This provides all the benefits of the combination and is THE *mudra* for peak digestion.

Timing: Practice this for 15-45 minutes every day (followed by 5-15 minutes of Prana *Mudra*), until the disease is cured.

39. Surya *Mudra*

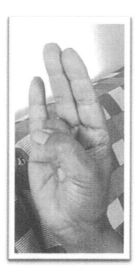

Instructions:
1. This *mudra* essentially reduces the earth element and increases the fire element within us.
2. Join the tip of your ring finger to the base of your thumb.
3. Gently press your thumb on the back of your ring finger.
4. Hold the remaining 3 fingers straight and lose.

Benefits: This *mudra* can dramatically increase the heat in your body, improve digestion and cure cold-related disorders. However, this is a *therapeutic mudra* and is hence restricted to 15-45 minutes of practice (required only until the disease is cured). Also, this *mudra* reduces the "heaviness" within us (by reducing the earth element) and is excellent for weight loss.

Timing: Practice this for 15-45 minutes every day (followed by 5-15 minutes of Prana *mudra*), until the disease is cured.

40. Shoonya *Mudra*

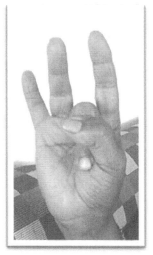

Instructions:
1. Join the tip of your middle finger to the base of your thumb.
2. Gently press your thumb on the back of your middle finger.
3. Hold the remaining 3 fingers straight and lose.

Benefits: This *mudra* essentially reduces the space or ether element within us and hence heals all hearing disorders and ear infections. It also provides an effective cure for Vertigo.

Timing: Practice this for 15-45 minutes every day (followed by 5-15 minutes of Prana *mudra*), until the disease is cured.

41. Kidney *Mudra*

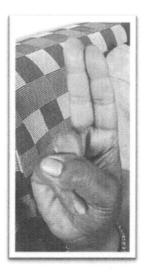

Instructions:
1. Join the tips of your ring and little fingers to the base of your thumb.
2. Gently press your thumb on the back of your these fingers.
3. Hold the remaining 3 fingers straight and lose.

Benefits: This *mudra* cures most Kidney disorders. It is also excellent to reduce water retention in the body, and regularize excess bleeding (during the menstrual cycle).

Timing: For chronic cases, practice this for 45 minutes every day (followed by 15 minutes of Prana *mudra*), until the disease is cured. For mild cases, practice this for 15 minutes every day (followed by 5 minutes of Prana *mudra*) until the disease is cured.

42. Linga *Mudra*

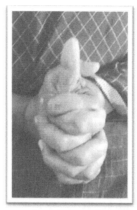

This is perhaps among the few *mudras* that needs to be practiced with both hands.

Instructions:
1. Join your palms together, facing each other.
2. Interlock your fingers so they form a steady grip. Raise your right thumb on top and keep it straight.

Benefits: This is an incredibly strong *Mudra* and increases the heat within our body. It is named so after the "Shiva Linga," a powerful manifestation of divine energy in Vedic tradition! This mudra improves our digestion and breathing, reduces our weight, relieves chest and nasal congestion and regularizes all activities of our naval center. However, this is a therapeutic *mudra* and should be practiced no longer than 15 minutes a day. It must also be combined with adequate consumption of liquids so the body is not overly heated.

Timing: 15 minutes every day.

43. Namaskara *Mudra*

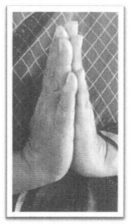

Instructions:
1. Join your palms together, palms facing each other and fingers pointed upward.
2. Carry humility within you and welcome the divinity in and around you!

Benefits: This is a welcoming *mudra* that you will find practiced by every spiritual Yogi!

This *mudra* increases the oneness we feel with others. With regular practice, this dissolves our ego as it constantly reminds us to recognize and connect with the divinity ever present amongst us.

Timing: As often and as long as you want!

SECTION – 3
THERAPEUTIC YOGA

9. Therapeutic Yoga

First, let me begin by telling you that there's no such thing as "therapeutic" Yoga (unlike Power Yoga or Yin Yoga). I use the term as a manner of speaking, to help you understand the therapeutic uses of combining Yogic techniques.

In this chapter, I briefly outline the optimum Yogic practice to deal with common ailments.

Yoga for Diabetes
Step 1 – *Asana:*
Practice 3-5 sets each of the *asanas* outlined below.
Vajrasana (Diamond pose) for 5 minutes
Paschimottasana (Seated forward bend pose)
Gomukhasana (Cow head pose)
Navasana (Boat pose)
Setu Bandhasana (Bridge pose)
Balasana (Child pose)

Step 2 – *Pranayama:*
1 set of Nadi Shodhana Pranayama (11 repetitions).
1-2 sets of Kapalbaati Pranayama (21 repetitions each).

Step 3 – *Mudra* with meditation:
Apana Vayu *mudra*, for 45 minutes.
Prana *mudra*, for 15 minutes.

Yoga to regularize (high) blood pressure
Step 1 – *Asana:*
Virasana for 2-5 minutes
Paschimottasana (Seated forward bend pose)
Adho Mukha Svanasana (Downward dog pose)
Setu Bandhasana (Bridge pose)
Makarasana (Crocodile pose)
Shavasana (Corpse pose)

Step 2 – *Pranayama:*
1 set of Nadi Shodhana Pranayama (11 repetitions).
Bhramari Pranayama for 2-5 minutes.

Step 3 – *Mudra* with meditation:

Apana Vayu *mudra*, for 45 minutes.
Prana *mudra*, for 15 minutes.

Yoga for improved digestion

Step 1 – Asana:
Practice 3-5 sets each of the *asanas* outlined below.
Vajrasana (Diamond pose) for 5-15 minutes
Paschimottasana (Seated forward bend pose)
Yoga Mudrasana (Psychic union pose)
12 repetitions of Suryanamaskar (Sun salutation)

Step 2 – Pranayama:
1 set of Nadi Shodhana Pranayama (11 repetitions).
3-5 sets of Kapalbaati Pranayama (21 repetitions each). With practice, you can increase this to 3 sets (of 50 repetitions each).

Step 3 – Mudra with meditation:
Vayu *Mudra* for 5 minutes.
Apana *Mudra*, for 45 minutes.
Prana *Mudra*, for 15 minutes.

Yoga for weight loss

Step 1 – Asana:
Practice 3-5 sets of any at least 5 asanas outlined for the body.
24 repetitions of Suryanamaskar (Sun salutation). You may start with a smaller number, based on your current fitness level and increase with practice.

Step 3 – Pranayama:
1 set of Nadi Shodhana Pranayama (11 repetitions).
5 sets of Kapalbaati Pranayama (50 repetitions each). If your fitness level doesn't support this, begin with 3 sets of 21 repetitions, and work up to the final number in 1 month.

Step 4 – Mudra with meditation:
Linga *Mudra* for 10 minutes.
Surya *Mudra*, for 10 minutes.
Prana *Mudra*, for 15 minutes.

Yoga for back pain

Step 1 – Asana:

Practice 3-5 sets each of the *asanas* outlined below.
Adho Mukha Svanasana (Downward dog pose)
Paschimottasana (Seated forward bend pose)
Chakravakasana (Cat cow stretch)
Setu Bandhasana (Bridge pose)
Balasana (Child pose)
6-12 repetitions of Suryanamaskar (Sun salutation)

Step 2 – *Pranayama*:
1 set of Nadi Shodhana Pranayama (11 repetitions).
Bhramari Pranayama for 2-5 minutes.

Step 3 – *Mudra* with meditation:
Vayu *Mudra* for 15-30 minutes.
Prana *Mudra*, for 10 minutes.

Yogic Kriyas for healing

Kriyas are a unique combination of Yogic body postures (*asana*) and breathing techniques (pranayama). Some will even use *bandhas* (Yogic body "locks") and hand postures (*mudra*). Together, *kriyas* can provide an effective cure to physical disease.

The science is simple. It recognizes physical disease as lack of "ease" within our body. This is caused, by a block in our body's energy system. By isolating the area of unease (through the body posture) and pumping energy into it (through breathing techniques), the block is removed. This automatically restores health.

While the practice of Kriyas is more suited to an advanced book on Yoga, I recommend exploring Kriyas using the link provided below. Here, you will find 108 unique Kriyas for common disorders and disease (with video and instructions). http://www.nithyananda.org/nithya-kriyas#gsc.tab=0

10. Next Steps and Conclusion

As you've perhaps discovered through this book, Yoga is a powerful lifestyle that encapsulates every part of us, to lead us from matter to consciousness. This science also blesses us with many uplifting benefits as we begin to discover and celebrate deeper dimensions of our being.

In this book, I've focused on the physical and mental wellness benefits of Yoga. In addition, I outline 2 incredible Yoga programs that can help you take a quantum leap in your journey with Yoga.

Nithya Yoga for an Inner Awakening!

His Holiness Paramahamsa Nithyananda, a young Enlightened Master from Southern India describes Yoga as *"not just adding more movement to life, but adding LIFE to movement"*! Through his exalted 21-day life program, Nithyananda uses several Vedic and Yogic techniques and modern life sciences to literally rewire a Yogic brain and help us re-create our desired future. Post the program, most participants report stunning health recoveries, remarkable material success and deeper clarity on life. Interesting facets of the program include consciously creating a Yogic body and Vedic mind, powerful and mystical initiation from a living Enlightened Master, third-eye awakening, increased awareness and plenty more. If these features fascinate you, do check out their official website at:
http://innerawakening.org/index-2.html
http://www.nithyananda.org/program/nithya-yoga-teacher-training

Authentic Rishikesh Yoga retreat at Parmarth Nikethan!

Rishikesh is often hailed as *the* phenomenal Yoga capital of the universe. And Rishikesh is neatly lined with some of the most authentic Yoga ashrams across the world, offering impressive programs for the curious beginner and the comfortably experienced teacher. Of this, the Parmath Nikethan ashram is a recognized source that allows visitors to enjoy a holistic and wholesome Yoga retreat. Each day culminates on the banks of the sacred Ganga, with the devotional "Ganga Arathi," a truly out-of-this-world experience. If this excites you, you can check out their official website at:
http://www.parmarth.org/
http://www.parmarth.org/yoga/2015-courses/

I gently encourage you to explore both as these are two distinct but enormously effective, *life-transforming* programs.

I thank you for staying with me on this magical journey! If you enjoyed this book, I'd greatly appreciate your review on Amazon.

Please Check Out My Other Books.

You can visit my Amazon Author Page to check out my other books including Crystal Healing For Beginners and Meditation For Beginners.
Please read and enjoy.

Thanks again

~ Diane Clarke